Going to Kindergarten (with food allergies)

WRITTEN BY DAVID PILCH.

ILLUSTRATED BY MARTIN PILCH
AND DAVID PILCH.

CONCEPT BY REBECCA LIFTMAN.

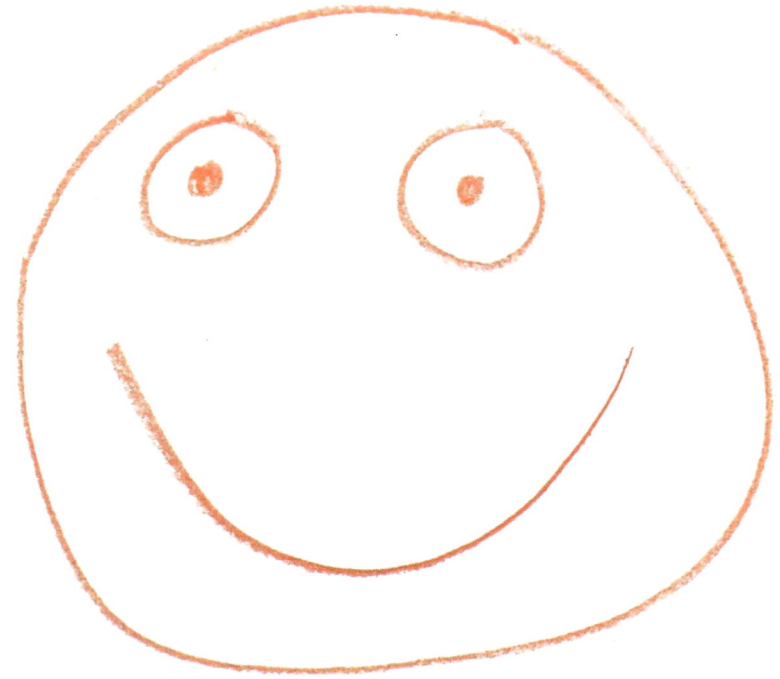

Hi. I'm Martin. I'm starting kindergarten this fall! That's exciting! And a little scary.

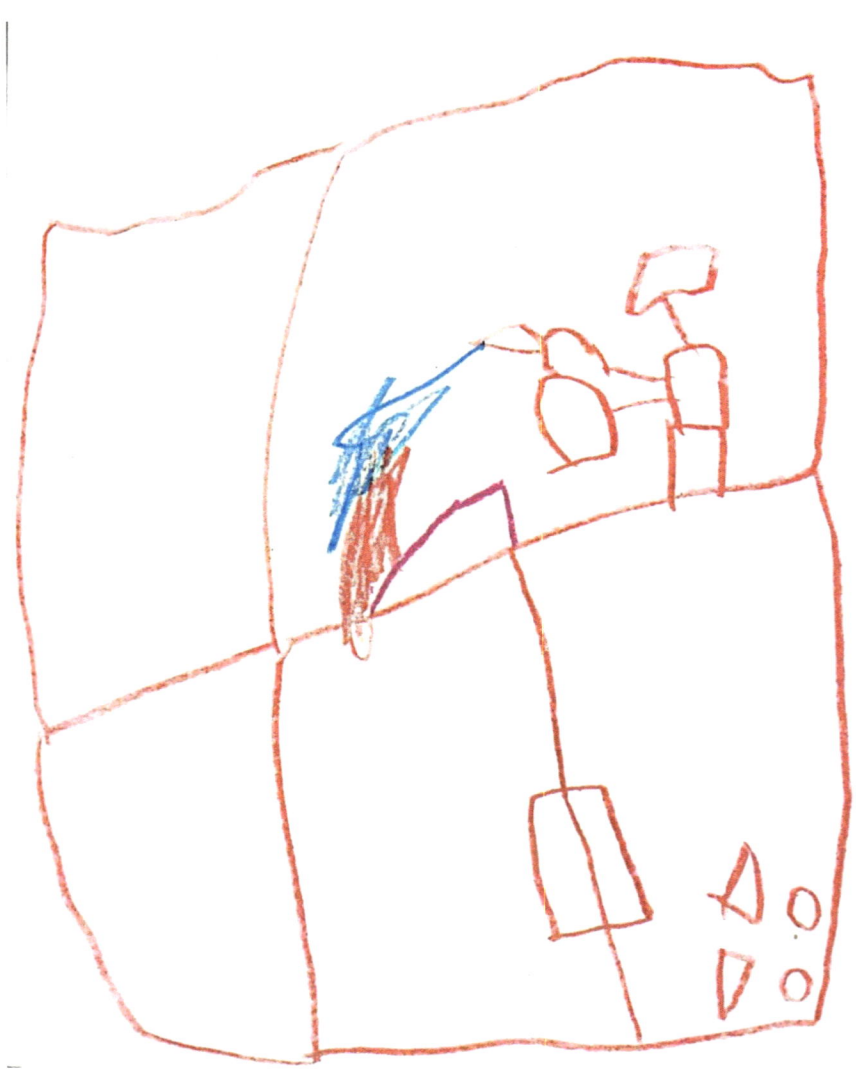

2

I like fire trucks, spaceships, construction vehicles, swimming, skiing, going on trips with my Dad and Mom, and story time at night before bed.

Here is a picture of me practicing my firefighting skills by using a fire extinguisher to put out a (pretend) fire.

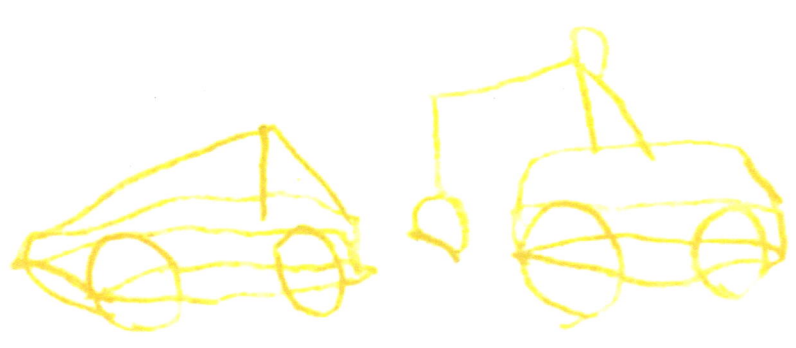

4

Here are some construction vehicles I drew!

I also have food allergies, so I have to be careful what I eat, and even what foods I touch.

I can't share food with other kids in kindergarten like I can in daycare, where all the food is allergy free.

I can't eat other people's food and I can't let them eat or touch my food.

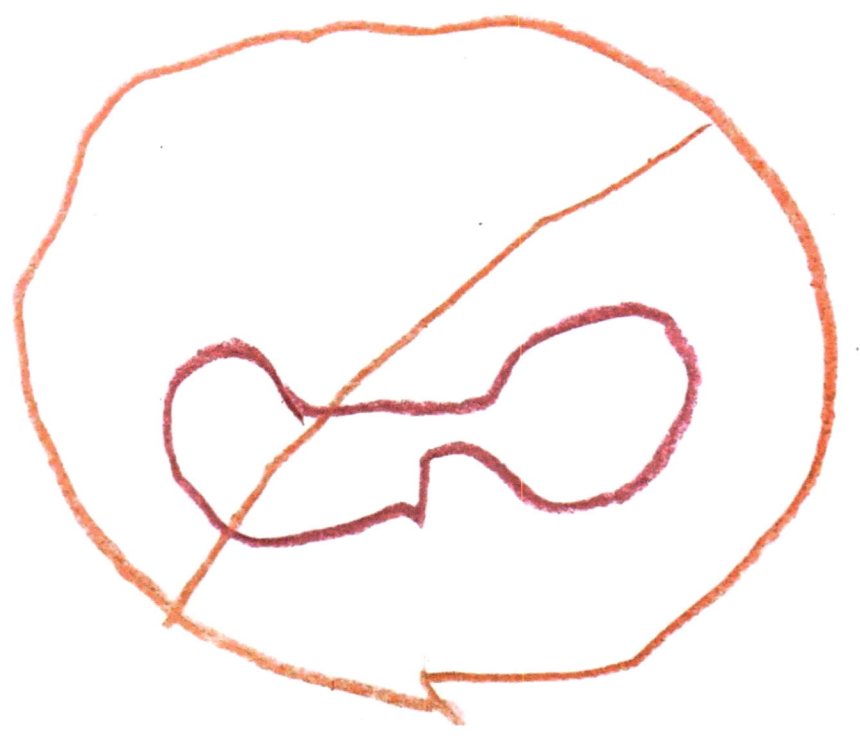

No Peanuts!

No tree nuts!

No Sesame seeds!

No fish!

Nothing made on mixed equipment!

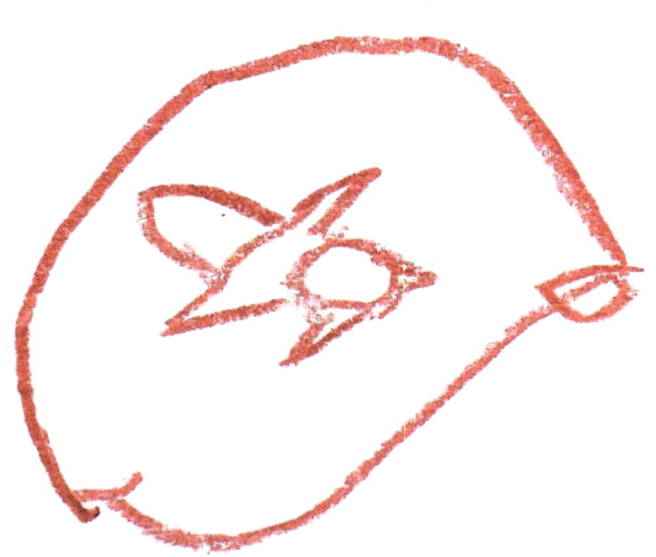

8

I wear my special super hero bracelet to kindergarten, which has a list of my allergies and the medicine to use if I have a reaction.

That way if I'm exposed to something, it can help a teacher or medical professional know what might be wrong with me if I'm having a reaction and can't talk.

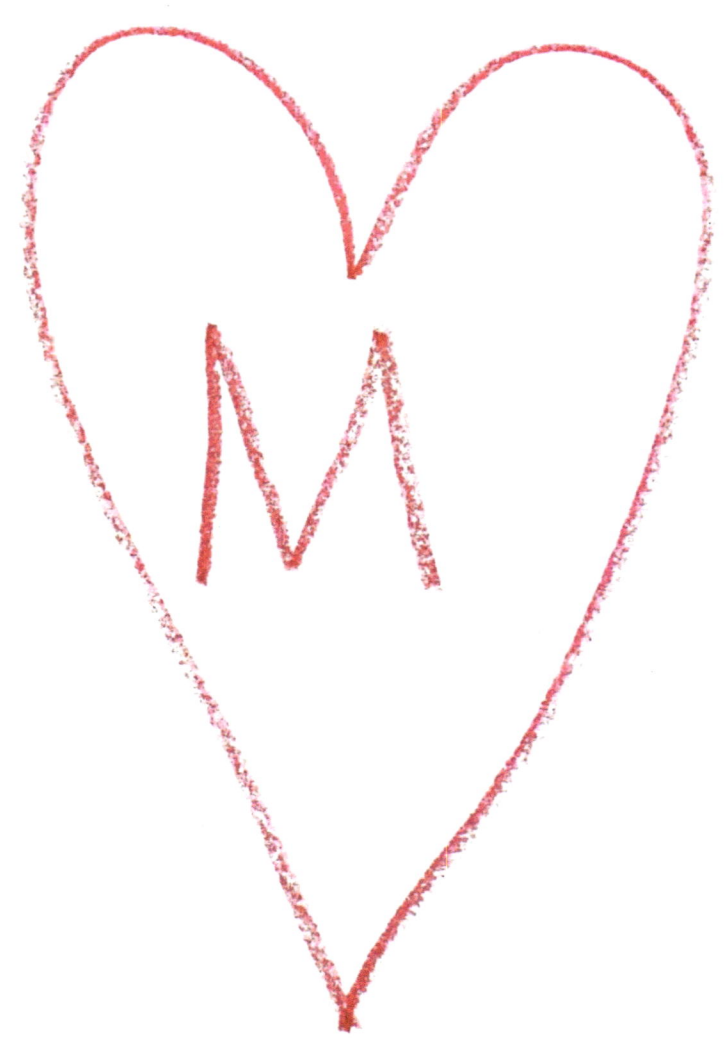

My parents love me so they are trying to teach me how to avoid foods to which I'm allergic in kindergarten, and what to do if I'm accidentally exposed to something to which I'm allergic.

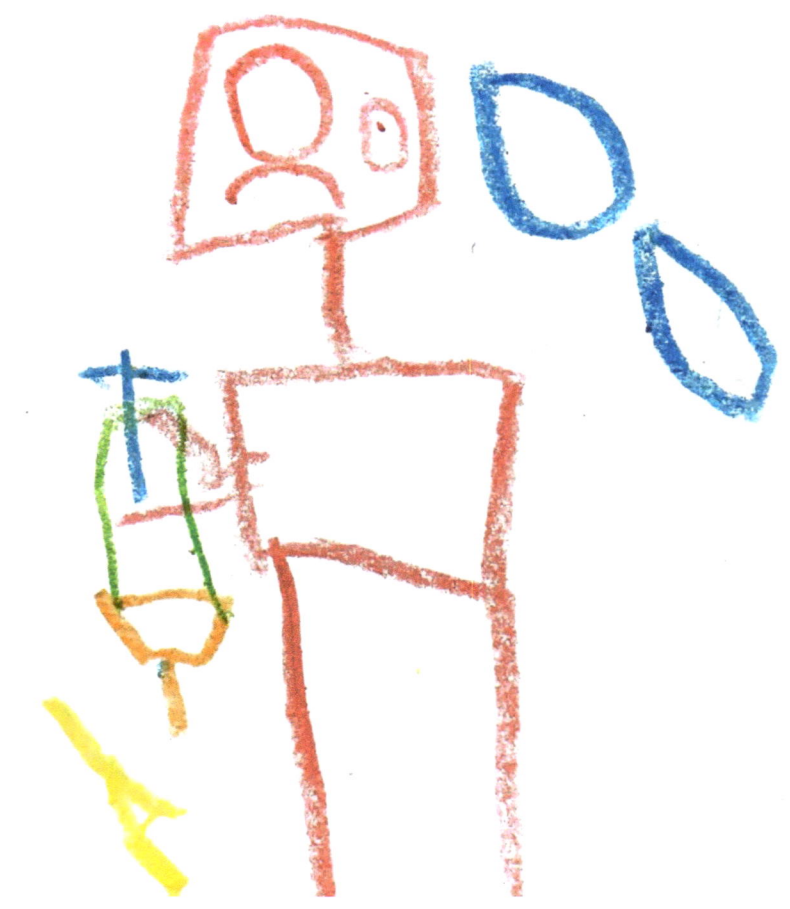

I have to carry and know how to use my own allergy medicine. It goes in my leg. One dose of epinephrine in my lunchbox, one in my backpack, and one in the nurse's office. I'd be sad if I needed it and didn't have it!

I'm a big kid now.

I'm going to kindergarten.

I have to start being responsible for my allergies.

I practice looking at and identifying foods to which I'm allergic with my Dad at the grocery store on Saturdays after

swimming.

I have to avoid foods to which I'm allergic.

I have to know how it feels when I am having a reaction.

I have to know how to give myself medicine if I have an allergy emergency.

I only use my medicine when I need it. It's not a toy. If I need it, I have to use it immediately.

You may have allergies that are different from mine.

You may not be allergic to anything at all.

Talk to your parents, and to your doctor, about what is best for you.

I'm just sharing what is best for me.

Will you help me avoid foods to which I'm allergic?

I'll give you lots of smiles, lots of laughter, great friendship, and tons of fun in return!

P.S., There are no naps in kindergarten like there are in daycare! That might take some getting used to! ?

www.ingramcontent.com/pod-product-compliance
Lightning Source LLC
Chambersburg PA
CBHW040329010626
45792CB00024B/2325